High Fructose Corn Syrup and the Fibromyalgia Connection

Fibromyalgia Recovery Handbook

by
Janice Lorigan

authorHOUSE®

AuthorHouse™
1663 Liberty Drive, Suite 200
Bloomington, IN 47403
www.authorhouse.com
Phone: 1-800-839-8640

First published by AuthorHouse 12/12/2007

ISBN: 978-1-4343-4976-7 (sc)

Library of Congress Control Number: 2007909064

*The advice contained in this book should be used only with
the approval of your own physician. Consult with a medical
doctor for all health problems, including fibromyalgia.*

*Printed in the United States of America
Bloomington, Indiana*

This book is printed on acid-free paper.

Dedication:

In gratitude to those who shared their stories,
those who believe in me and Google.

"The proof is in the pudding!"

Table of Contents

Introduction .... *ix*

Chapter I
What Fibromyalgia Is *1*

Chapter II
Your Recovery Guidelines *5*

Chapter III
Corn Syrup and High Fructose Corn Syrup *9*

Chapter IV
*Digestion, Metabolism, and High Fructose
Corn Syrup* *13*

Chapter V
*Metabolism, High Fructose Corn Syrup, and
Fibromyalgia* *17*

Chapter VI
Fascia, Pain, and Central Nervous System *21*

Chapter VII
Fatigue and Energy *27*

Chapter VIII
Food for Fibromyalgics.. 29

Chapter IX
Other Issues... 33

Chapter X
Moving Forward.. 37

About the Author 41

Introduction

This book if for those with fibromyalgia who are searching for answers. My intent is to provide you with sufficient guidance to support your steady and speedy recovery. Although some of the contents seem a little technical, they are needed to adequately address the following:

Causes of Fibromyalgia
Metabolism and Its Relationship to Fibromyalgia
Treatment for Fibromyalgia

I struggled with selecting an appropriate title. I chose "High Fructose Corn Syrup and the Fibromyalgia Connection" over "High Fructose Corn Syrup is a Low-Down Disingenuous, Little Snake in the Grass."

Treatment will not require any medication, prescriptions, therapies, surgery, or unhealthy practices. Like millions of others, you may have already tried pain-reducers, muscle relaxants, chiropractors, anti-depressants, chelating agents, water therapy, and/or meditation. Although some of those measures provide a small amount of relief, none of them address the basic causes of fibromyalgia. Therefore, all of those treatments fall short.

I am honored to provide you with the startling and cheerful news. Not only will you have the power to avoid most of the pain, achiness, fatigue, and desperation of fibromyalgia, you will conquer feelings of bewilderment and helplessness. Your overall health may benefit also. Chapters two and eight include specific guidelines needed for recovery. The other chapters explain the effect of high fructose corn syrup on metabolism and body chemistry.

Janice Lorigan
October 5, 2007

Chapter I
What Fibromyalgia Is

Fibromyalgia is a syndrome of symptoms that wax and wane. The term itself means pain in the muscles and fibrous (connective) tissue. Although the term was rarely used before 1980, many of us have endured painful bouts of fibromyalgia since the 1970s.

The symptoms of fibromyalgia are many. The primary symptoms are pain in the muscles and connective tissue, fatigue, un-restorative or lack of deep sleep, and achiness. Other common symptoms are irritable bowel syndrome; increased sensitivity to touch, pain, or heat; headaches and neck aches; depression or catastrophic thinking; and stiffness.

Many more females than males have been diagnosed with fibromyalgia. However, this affliction strikes males and females, young and old. There are millions suffering with fibromyalgia in the U.S., Canada, and European countries.

Fibromyalgia is neither contagious nor fatal (maybe its only positive descriptions). Fibromyalgia causes chronic pain, achiness, and fatigue. The discomfort is significant, debilitating, and difficult to relieve.

Medical personnel have been perplexed by the complaints of pain because of the lack of observable injuries to the body, lack of evidence of an infectious disease, and lack of evidence of cancer or organ malfunction coupled with the lack of scientific studies that have identified the causes. Fibromyalgia does not fit any of the established medical models. Frequently fibromyalgics look like they are healthy and robust because of the disguised nature of the causes and the good appearance of the fibromyalgic. Some doctors and others assume that the problems are psychogenic or psychosomatic in origin.

Fibromyalgia is not caused by psychological, mental, or emotional problems. Your illness and pain have a biochemical basis. The problems stem from dysfunction in your liver, intestines, connective tissues, central nervous system, and fascia. This dysfunction is caused by chemicals from the environment that confound and distress metabolic processes at the cellular level.

Some symptoms of fibromyalgia overlap with the symptoms of Gulf-War syndrome and chronic fatigue syndrome. Future research may reveal whether the three maladies are "cousins." Fibromyalgia, Gulf-War syndrome, and chronic fatigue were all named at the end of the twentieth century.

Causes of medical diseases and disorders are grouped usually into one of the following categories:
- Poisons
- Infectious Diseases
- Cancer
- Allergies
- Metabolic Disorders

Because of its temporary nature and because of its dependence upon outside (environmental) influences, fibromyalgia has similar characteristics to those of poisons and allergies. However, the involvement of the endocrine system of the fibromyalgic closely matches diseases characterized as "metabolic disorders."

Metabolic disorders have some characteristics that do not apply to fibromyalgia. Most metabolic disorders have strong genetic components (Tay-Sachs, sickle cell anemia). Many metabolic disorders result, in part, from organ dysfunction or damage. (Examples include pancreatic dysfunction with diabetes or liver impairment in fatty liver disease.) Typically a genetic defect is blamed for the abnormal behavior of digestive enzymes. The intermittent nature of fibromyalgia and its lack of an established genetic component disqualify fibromyalgia from the metabolic disorder group.

As further explanation, consider this analogy. If someone swallows a large amount of poison (more than the liver and endocrine system can neutralize or dispose of), he or she will become very ill, often with violent body reactions and severe (or even fatal) interruptions to body functions. This acute dysfunction following the ingestion of poison is not blamed on a physical disorder or malfunction of the body. The poison is blamed, not the body.

Fibromyalgia requires a new classification. An appropriate title might be "induced metabolism dysfunction" or "confounded metabolism."

Chapter II
Your Recovery Guidelines

Later chapters contain explanations of why you need to make some changes. This chapter is a succinct guideline of what you must do to reduce fibromyalgic symptoms and obtain greater control over your body. (You can begin recovery prior to finishing the book.)

The offensive substances are contained in the beverages you drink, foods you eat, and sometimes the air that you breathe.

DO NOT

- Eat food products that contain high fructose corn syrup, corn syrup, crystalline fructose, or corn syrup solids.
- Inhale wet fingernail polish fumes

- Inhale pesticides, insecticides, fumigants, or malathion (commercial or home-use products)
- Drink liquids in which any of the ingredients contains more than 5 percent pesticides
- Drink liquids that contain high fructose corn syrup (HFCS), corn syrup*, crystalline fructose, or corn syrup solids
- Eat rice**

*Old-time, regular corn syrup does not disturb metabolic processes for most people. However, many manufacturers are still using the terms *high fructose corn syrup* and *corn syrup* interchangeably.

**Rice, without excessive amounts of arsenic, is a wonderful, nutritious food. Unfortunately, rice absorbs arsenic from the soil. (Soil of many agricultural areas of the U.S. and other countries has elevated levels of arsenic.)

DO

- Read ingredient levels on food and beverage containers
- Err on the side of caution when eating out
- Stock your pantry or kitchen cupboard with organic crackers, cookies, and cereals. Stock your refrigerator with fresh fruits and vegetables

- Wash fruits and vegetables thoroughly
- When possible, drink filtered water
- Drink organic milk and organic juice
- If you are a wine drinker, seek out organic wine
- Eat a balanced diet (that excludes HFCS)

The foods listed above are specific for those with fibromyalgia. Of course, other medical conditions require different dietary restrictions. Therefore, check with your own physician regarding dietary additions and deletions.

Organic rice may have minimal amounts of pesticides. However, it may contain an excessive amount of arsenic. If rice is grown on acreage where cotton was grown previously, there can be a heavy concentration of arsenic in the soil. (Strong pesticides containing arsenic were used to kill boll weevils on cotton fields.) When rice is grown in the same soil, at a later time, the arsenic is absorbed into the rice as it grows. The levels of arsenic in tested rice have alarmed scientists.

The word *natural* on food products does not promise minimal levels of pesticides or the exclusion of high fructose corn syrup. The word *organic* on the label is a guarantee that no ingredient in the product has a higher concentration of pesticides than five percent. To date, I have never seen the words *high fructose corn syrup* on any food product labeled organic.

Chapter III
Corn Syrup and High Fructose Corn Syrup

Grinding and milling corn to produce food have been around for centuries. Corn, corn meal, and cornstarch are important components of many meals. Corn is a nutritious, dietary staple.

In the mid-1800s, a method of acid conversion was applied to cornstarch to produce a sweetener (corn syrup). Hydrolysis is the term used to describe this conversion process. This acid method of converting cornstarch to sweet corn syrup has been used for more than a hundred years.

In the late 1960s, an enzymatic method of conversion of corn syrup was developed that increased the amount of fructose in the syrup and changed the proportion of fructose to glucose.

Some of the glucose of the corn syrup is converted to fructose. Two or three separate stages of the conversion process require the application of enzymes. Today it is estimated that high fructose corn syrup is 40 to 90 percent fructose.

The newer, manufactured high fructose corn syrup is sweeter and more soluble than regular corn syrup. In the early 1970s, a faster method for producing high fructose corn syrup was developed. Sweet high fructose corn syrup was added to the American diet by way of a great variety of commercial foods and beverages. Food manufacturers appreciate the attractive features of high fructose corn syrup. These agreeable components are:

- Sweetness
- Solubility
- Transportability
- Contribution to food consistency
- Stability at various temperatures
- Longer shelf-life
- Humectant properties (retains moisture)

The amount of high fructose corn syrup in processed foods has greatly increased in the last three decades. Currently the number of products that include HFCS as an ingredient has climbed into the thousands. Yogurt, baked goods, crackers, fruit drinks, soda, pancake syrup, jams, ketchup, energy bars, lunch meats, cold cereals, canned fruits, salad dressings, hamburger buns, hotdog buns, and pre-packaged bread, cake, and muffins include high fructose corn syrup.

Non-fibromyalgic consumers seem to metabolize high fructose corn syrup with no noticeable unpleasant effects. Fibromyalgics experience negative effects after eating or drinking high fructose corn syrup. (However, the effects are not immediate.) It is difficult for the fibromyalgic to make the connection between the pain and the HFCS, because the problems may not occur until one or two days after ingestion of HFCS.

Chapter IV
Digestion, Metabolism, and High Fructose Corn Syrup

Digestion and metabolism are chemical processes that take food and beverages into the body, break the materials down into smaller substances, and convert the substances into nutrients and energy for cells. Enzymes and hydrolic acid begin to work in the mouth to break the food into smaller, dissolvable components. In the stomach a variety of other enzymes prepare molecules and liquids for assimilation and metabolism.

High fructose corn syrup does not cause problems for the digestive process. However, high fructose corn syrup is challenging and strife-ridden for the metabolism of fibromyalgics.

Metabolism begins with life and continues until death. Metabolism and life are inseparable. Metabolism is the process of providing nutrients that aid in repair, cellular activity, organ and gland functioning, blood circulation, activity of hormones and neurotransmitters, motor activities, and thinking. Metabolism begins in the stomach and continues into the rest of the body. Complex, chemical processes work continuously in the small intestine, liver, glands, and cells.

The journey of high fructose corn syrup into the body reminds us of the fable of the Trojan horse. The Greeks conquered Troy by hiding inside a huge, wooden horse. The horse was given to the Trojans as a gift. Once inside the gates of Troy, the Greek soldiers snuck out of the wooden horse at night, surprised and attacked the Trojans, and conquered Troy.

High fructose corn syrup tastes like food in the mouth and digests like food in the stomach. It is palatable and is accepted by the body as it travels through the mouth, esophagus, and stomach. Once high fructose corn syrup is consumed, it spends several hours in the digestive process (like food). (Its Trojan horse is being a substance that tastes and acts like food.) As metabolism begins, the body discovers the deception. Part of the high fructose syrup is toxic to fibromyalgics.

High fructose corn syrup is an anomaly to the metabolic process.

Chapter V
Metabolism, High Fructose Corn Syrup, and Fibromyalgia

Metabolism is continuous, but toxic or ambiguous substances that enter into the body can stall or cripple parts or metabolism. A depressed metabolism impacts the enzymes, hormones, and neurotransmitters—all vital for cell activity (growth, repair, energy, and communication between cells, glands, organs, and the central nervous system).

High fructose corn syrup is sweet and non-irritating during digestion as it travels easily from the mouth, through the esophagus, and into the stomach. For the fibromyalgic, problems begin to occur during metabolism, when the digested mixture is being prepared for assimilation and distribution.

Part of the high fructose corn syrup is solidly fructose, part is glucose, and part is a chemically manipulated fructose that used to be glucose. An involved process of enzymatic applications and heating and cooling at different stages of the HFCS manufacturing process convert glucose into fructose. However, the metabolic chemical processes in the cells can re-affect the new fructose.

Enzymes can change the shape and consistency of a substance. For example, when you add hot water to a dry gelatin mixture, the mixture and water blend together into a very fluid state. Then you add cold water, mix, and refrigerate. Within a few hours, the gelatin has become more solid and rubbery. The gelatin can no longer be poured like a liquid. However, the gelatin can revert into a more liquid state if it is left out on a hot day. Heat and cold can affect and re-affect enzymatic action. In addition to heat and cold changing enzymatic actions, so does adding a different enzyme. (There are an estimated two thousand different enzymes in the human body.) Gelatin gels very well if peaches or pears are added to the mix. In contrast, pineapple contains its own enzymes that will interfere with or prevent the enzymes of the gelatin from making it gel. (Most gelatin boxes have a note of advice that warns the cook about trying to include pineapple.)

If the chemically created fructose has made its way into cells throughout the body and has now reverted back into glucose, the cells will begin to combine with oxygen and ATP to create energy (or at least try to). If the chemically created fructose has remained fructose, it must return to the liver for metabolism. (All fructose is metabolized in the liver.) Other sugars, including glucose, are not restricted to the liver for metabolism. Cells throughout the body need tremendous quantities of glucose. The mitochondria of the tissue cells use oxygen and glucose (not fructose) to produce energy. The energy is supplied to the neuron for all the life-sustaining activities of the cell.

The unique fructose component of high fructose corn syrup confuses the metabolic processes and exhausts the intestines and liver with the burdens of unstable fructose or modified glucose (or both). Both organs and neurotransmitters (hormones) are affected.

Serotonin and dopamine are neurotransmitters that contribute to feelings of contentment and well-being. Canadian researchers have found that during pain, the dopamine levels in fibromyalgics are significantly lower than the dopamine levels in non-fibromyalgics. (It isn't clear whether the dopamine lessens prior to the pain or whether the pain contributes to the lower levels of dopamine.)

The literature states that approximately 95 percent of serotonin (considered the "happy" hormone) is produced in the intestines. In fibromyalgics the low levels of serotonin contribute to depression and catastrophic or negative thinking. As long as the intestines are overtaxed with the abnormal glucose/fructose metabolism problem, serotonin production may be very depressed.

Enzymes are proteins and chemical catalysts. There are numerous types of enzymes. Each type of enzyme aids in the process of one type of molecule (or, at the most, a couple types of those molecules). Enzymes influence the speed of metabolism and play powerful roles in the metabolic process.

The pancreas (gland of the endocrine system) manufactures enzymes. One of the important roles of the enzyme is to remove toxins from the body. Poisons decrease the production of enzymes. Therefore, a lower level of enzymes makes ridding the body of toxins more difficult, and the higher level of toxins suppresses the production of much needed enzymes. Some of the work of removing poisons and toxins from the body occurs in the small intestine. Similar to the situation with the production of serotonin, the decrease in the production of enzymes may also result from the burden on the intestines because of the glucose/fructose dilemma.

Chapter VI
Fascia, Pain, and Central Nervous System

Researchers and fibromyalgics have confirmed the connection between fibromyalgia and fascia. Fascia is a stretchy web existing all over the body. It lies just below the skin. The fascia surrounds internal organs, the brain, toes and fingers, limbs, neck, and the complete musculoskeletal system. The fascia helps to hold the body together, sustains the physique, and supports and separates organs and muscles.

To date there is a sparse amount of literature regarding the chemistry of the fascia. In the last decade, the scientific community has given more attention to this very important connective tissue structure.

Fascia that is in optimal condition is very elastic and moves easily over the musculoskeletal systems. The fascia is made up of connective tissue cells that contain fibroblasts and a sticky substance. The sticky substance and the fibroblast work together to protect internal organs; support the head, muscles, and bones; and stretch and contract to facilitate movement and physical activity.

The connective tissue of the lumbar (torso) of the body consists of cells that have a higher (or denser) concentration of fibroblasts than the connective tissue on the arms and legs. Therefore, impaired fascia of the fibromyalgic becomes tighter and more immobile in the neck, upper back, shoulders, and lower back. A lower concentration of fibroblasts in the legs and arms allows for less tightness and restriction.

At times the fascia of fibromyalgics contains and restrains the muscle, ligaments, and tendons too tightly. Manipulation of the fascia with massage, acupuncture, or acupressure provides some comfort.

There are no answers regarding what occurs in fascia to hamper its flexibility or stretchiness and then what occurs that allows fascia to regain its stretchiness. My hypothesis is that the enzymes—used originally to change some glucose to fructose during the creation of HFCS—are assimilated into the small intestine and cells during metabolism. The body does not need these strange enzymes, and the body acts to excrete the extra enzymes out of the body through the pores of the skin (similar to excretion of toxins through sweat and the pores or the excretion of some chemicals of garlic).

To reach the pores of the skin, the HFCS enzymes must pass (from the cells of the tissue, ligament, and muscles) through the fascia. The strange enzymes reach the fascia fibroblasts and jelly-like substance and reacts with the natural enzymes of the fascia. This adverse chemical reaction stiffens the fascia and inhibits the stretchiness until the HFCS enzymes are expelled from the fascia. (Refer to chapter five for the explanation of gelatin and pineapple enzymes.)

Unfortunately, while the fascia is stiff and contracted, the body feels pain and achiness. The thin, stretchy web, called fascia, is forceful enough to crowd and inhibit the musculoskeletal system; Recovery for some fibromyalgics requires additional sleep time. The intestines, liver, endocrine system, and cells work very hard and use a significant amount of energy to rid the body of high fructose corn syrup chemicals. Pain and fatigue are primary symptoms of fibromyalgia.

Most of the tissues of the body contain pain receptors. (There are a few exceptions—brain, parts of the intestines.) The ligaments, tendons, and muscles contain millions of pain receptors. The pain receptors, located throughout the body, connect with the central nervous system so that the brain is given a clear message. The message of pain is, "You've got problems!"

The thalamus is an area of the brain that is made up of neurons (nerve cells). The thalamus, as part of the central nervous system, plays a part in neural coordination and pain processing. There is evidence of a lower level of activity in the thalamus of fibromyalgics. In addition, pain inhibitory pathways and pain facilitatory pathways in the central nervous system of fibromyalgics appear to behave differently than those of non-fibromyalgics. (It isn't known whether the pathways of fibromyalgics are permanently abnormal or behave irregularly just during periods of pain.) The differences in the activity of the central nervous system may account for the disproportionate degree of pain felt and reported.

The pain and achiness of fibromyalgics results, in part, from contracted fascia restricting and applying pressure to the muscles, tendons, ligaments, and organs. Abnormal processing in the pathways of the central nervous system may exacerbate the degree of pain.

Chemicals in high fructose corn syrup, pesticides, and insecticides burden metabolism. These chemicals negatively affect the neurotransmitters, hormones, and fascia and slow the speed by which pancreatic enzymes and the liver can rid the body of toxins. Protect your body by being aware of what you are eating and drinking, reading ingredient labels and avoiding pesticides and high fructose corn syrup.

Chapter VII
Fatigue and Energy

Fatigue is a handicap of nearly all who suffer from fibromyalgia. Many complain that even after hours of sleep, they still feel tired or even exhausted. Some sleep for a day or more and wake up every so often only to return to sleep after an hour or so of wakefulness. Climbing a flight or two of stairs seems to require almost more energy than the fibromyalgic has.

Neither explanations of physical exhaustion nor explanations of emotional exhaustion account for the fatigue of fibromyalgics. The fatigue is unrelated to strenuous exercise. Fibromyalgia fatigue results from a confounded metabolism and insufficient energy production in cells. Cells need glucose to produce energy for the body. (Unlike glucose, fructose has a very limited part in energy production.)

The mitochondria (the "powerhouse" of the cells) produce energy, and the mitochondria need a constant supply of oxygen and glucose. Fructose can be metabolized only in the cells of the liver. Glucose is metabolized in cells in all tissues and organs throughout the body. High fructose corn syrup (40 to 90 percent fructose, approximately) overtaxes the liver. The mitochondria of the cells may not be able to use abnormal glucose that is now more closely related to fructose (or somewhere in between the two).

Toxins in the body also decrease cellular function. Arsenic (found in many pesticides and insecticides) disturbs glucose metabolism. Slowed and disturbed metabolism may contribute to the overall feeling of fatigue. In addition, as discussed previously, the cells may be producing less energy because of an inadequate amount of glucose or an unusable form of glucose.

Chapter VIII
Food for Fibromyalgics

Always read ingredient labels! Manufacturers have the option of changing the ingredients. If a food product states that it is organic, there should be only a minimal amount of pesticides and no high fructose corn syrup.

Below is a list of acceptable foods

Fresh Vegetables (well-washed)
Pizza
Lamb and Pork
Beans
Frozen Vegetables
Oats
Fresh fruit (well-washed)
Organic cold cereal
Frozen fruit
Organic peanut butter

Eggs
Gravy
Cheese
Organic maple syrup
Organic milk
Organic cookies and crackers
Butter
Mustard
Organic fruit juice
Pickle relish
Chicken, turkey, and duck
Organic jams and jellies
Home-baked breads, cakes
Salmon and ocean fish
Puddings (box)
Cakes and cookies (made from scratch)
Flour tortillas
Some canned soups (organic)
Pasta and noodles
Some canned beans (organic)
organic spaghetti sauces
Some canned fruits
Jell-O and gelatin
Organic ice cream*
Nuts
Some candies**
Pickles (check label)
Tea Unsweetened
Olive oil
applesauce
Coconut oil
Honey
Granulated and powdered cane sugar

*At this writing, Breyer's natural strawberry, cherry vanilla, and butter pecan ice creams contain no high fructose corn syrup.

**At this writing, Hershey's chocolate kisses and some specialty chocolate bars contain no HFCS.

A note about bread: It is difficult to find pre-packaged bread that does not contain high fructose corn syrup. However, if the grocery store has a bakery, the bakery may have breads that are free of high fructose corn syrup.

Eating out is a special challenge. It is easy to forget that marinara pasta sauces, breads used for sandwiches and toast, bagels, Worcestershire sauce, most salad dressings, bottled fruit drinks, and fruit pies contain HFCS.

Chapter IX
Other Issues

Fibromyalgia is unique, and its causes do not fall into the current medical models. Earlier literature details conditions called fibromyositis and fibrositis. They are characterized by restricted movement, like fibromyalgia. However, both fibromyositis and fibrositis are described as resulting from injury or inflammation to the muscles, unlike fibromyalgia.

Fibromyalgia (the term and reports of its symptoms) did not exist before highly processed foods containing high fructose corn syrup were commonly included in the American diet. It is difficult to ignore the parallel between the increase in the number of products containing high fructose corn syrup and the increase in the number of people diagnosed with fibromyalgia.

Some researchers believe that the strong toxins in pesticides have weakened the metabolism and the endocrine system. Subsequently, the weakened system cannot process efficiently added toxins or abnormal substances.

More than 90 percent of the population does not complain of fibromyalgia. As with other diseases (shingles, tuberculosis, strokes, macular degeneration, influenza—to name a few), the explanations of why some become ill and others remain unaffected are general. Weakened immune systems, bio-chemical flaws, exposure to environmental factors, infections, injury, nutritional deficiencies, and/or genetic predispositions are all reasons that are frequently proposed.

Many more females than males are diagnosed with fibromyalgia. Less than 20 percent of fibromyalgics are male. To date there are no validated answers that explain the disparate rates in the population. Males and females have basic bio-chemical differences, besides the obvious differences of genitalia and hair growth patterns. In general the muscles and brains of males have larger masses than those of females. Females also have a longer intestinal system and more pain receptors than do males (especially in the skin). Testosterone and estrogen (hormones) are in very different proportion. Women are affected by the forceful hormonal fluctuations related to menstruation, ovulation, pregnancy, childbirth, and menopause.

Arsenic, a poison and chemical element, has been established as an endocrine disruptor. (Future research will identify other chemicals with the same damaging potential.) Endocrine disruptors interfere with the hormones and body functions. There are currently more than seventy thousand chemicals used commercially. (Examples include cleaning solvents, oven cleaners, paint thinners, gasoline, plastics, and pesticides.) We have yet to see how many more chemicals of the seventy thousand will someday be identified as endocrine disruptors. Additional research on the endocrine system and metabolism may provide information on the disparate rates of fibromyalgia in males and females.

Chapter X
Moving Forward

This book is of value only if it works for you. Since a change in diet is required, you may want to explain to your doctor that you will be avoiding all high fructose corn syrup and as much pesticide residue as possible.

Hopefully, you understand that the functions of all systems and organs of the body are very closely linked. Chemicals, enzymes, and hormones facilitate functioning and speed or slow the connections. There are thousands of chemicals -- man-made and natural. Many chemicals seriously threaten our health, if ingested or inhaled.

My dream is that in the next few weeks, you are nearly pain-free and most of your achiness and fatigue have disappeared. Many fresh fruits and vegetables and processed foods have a small amount of pesticide residue. It is prudent to minimize the amount consumed by washing produce carefully and by purchasing organic beverages and products.

Each of us has a unique bio-chemical makeup, and the severity of fibromyalgia varies in each of us. Read all ingredient labels, exercise caution when eating out, and eliminate high fructose corn syrup from your diet. The reward for your diligence will be less pain and fatigue and more good days for a fuller life.

Moving forward and being grateful for small blessings is our best course of action. The manufacturers of high fructose corn syrup introduced a substance into our diets that contains no vitamins or minerals. In addition, high fructose corn syrup added to food and beverages compromises our health and well-being and depletes our energy.

Read all ingredient labels and reject any foods with high fructose corn syrup, crystalline fructose, corn syrup solids, or any other euphemisms that mean the same thing. Keep some distance between yourself and pesticides, powerful cleaning products, and pest fumigants.

Best wishes for a speedy recovery, healthier diet, and brighter future. Please provide me with feedback on your own experiences.

jlorigan@pacbell.net

October 2007

About the Author

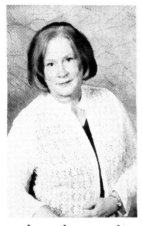

Janice Lorigan grew up in Ohio, the oldest child of Walter Finley, a railroad train dispatcher, and Emma who taught first grade. In 1962, the six Finleys moved to Southern California. Janice's awareness of the unrest and tragedies of the sixties contributed to her life-long interests in racial and gender equality, socio-economic justice, consumer rights, and product safety.

In her twenties, Ms. Lorigan married and worked as a secretary at George Washington University and the National Academy of Sciences in Washington, D.C. Her son was born in Alexandria, Virginia. After relocating to Southern California and after the birth of her daughter, she returned to college. She earned her B.A. and M.A.

Degrees from California State University, Los Angeles.

More than twenty years were devoted to child rearing and working as an analyst, specialist, and recruiter in the field of human resources. Janice has called South Pasadena her home since 1973. Her son, daughter, son-in-law, and two grandchildren reside there also. Our author finds joy in learning, laughter, great movies and books, and playing with her two best buddies -- Josephine and James (Grandchildren, of course).

Lightning Source UK Ltd.
Milton Keynes UK
05 June 2010

155201UK00001B/7/A

9 781434 349767